Atha
Sally-Shakti Willow

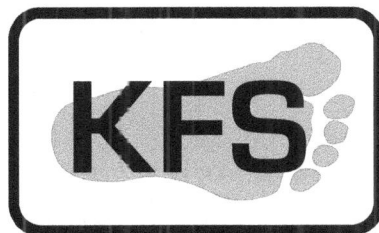

KFS

NEWTON-LE-WILLOWS

Published in the United Kingdom in 2019
by The Knives Forks And Spoons Press,
51 Pipit Avenue,
Newton-le-Willows,
Merseyside,
WA12 9RG.

ISBN 978-1-912211-43-2

Acknowledgements:

I am grateful for the unending support of Joe Evans, Kim West, David West, Peter West,
Joy West, Hermione Watson, Rob Watson, Marnie Padmai, Sarah Marie, Diana Sampson,
Morgan Khalsa, Lyn Core, Stephen Poole & all my family and friends who have shared
this vision with me.

This collection was created as part of my PhD in Utopian Poetics at the University of
Westminster. Grateful thanks to my supervisors John Beck, Georgina Colby, and Kristen
Kreider (at Goldsmiths), and to Leigh Wilson, Matthew Morrison and Alex Warwick.

Working with Alec Newman at Knives, Forks & Spoons Press has been a joy for which I
am extremely thankful. The sensitive attention both of Alec and of Scott Thurston in
reading and preparing these poems has helped to make this book what it is.

Joe Evans' work on the cover design and internal doodling, as ever, demonstrates his
intimate understanding of my words and work.

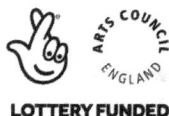

LOTTERY FUNDED

Supported using public funding by
**ARTS COUNCIL
ENGLAND**

For Lyn, who taught me that Atha is also 'utter'

Contents

Part 1:
Writing Utopia Now

WRITING UTOPIA NOW

Atha yogānuśāsanam

Āsana : posture=position=thesis

      pose, position [thesis].   Every yoga pose a thesis.

Atha : Now

           Now, an exposition of yoga

    yoga : *yuj*=yoke=union

NOW YOGA THESIS

[Now: thesis of union]

communion / non-alienation / non-oppression / utopia/n

Utopian poetics is the performance of a relationship of non-alienation between reader and writer, listener and speaker. This relationship exists in/as the poem's performance. The poem may be performed visually on the page, materially in the book, or physically as a spoken text. All of these performances of a poem – and others – may happen simultaneously.

WHERE IS THE POEM LOCATED?

WHERE IS THE POEM ENACTED?

WHERE DOES THE POEM LIVE?

The poem is located in the space between the writer and the receiver of the text; it is enacted in the [sub]vocalising, breathing body of the reader while reading, the writer while writing, the listener while listening, the speaker while speaking. In the writing/reading/speaking/listening/poem/text/breathing: The poem lives. In this space of non-alienation, the poem performs a utopian poetics by which the reader and the writer are not alienated from one another, but are brought into relationship by the poem as it is performed. ***Poems need readers to live. Poems need writers to give them form.*** In this space of non-oppression neither the writer nor the reader is superior nor subordinate. In this space of non-alienation and non-oppression, the writer-speaker-reader-listener is/are **intersubjective**. Living/reading/breathing [in] the poem as the poem is living/writing/breathing [in] us. Utopian poetics brings writereaders into a communional space of presence, which is both no-place and perfect-place (*e/u/topia*), where we may experience ourselves as simultaneously both embodied subjects and intersubjective beings. ***Tat twam asi***. You Are That. Self-realisation as both embodied and intersubjective. Non-alienated both from ourselves and from others. This is the essence of the utopian. Utopian poetics ***performs*** this, it does not describe. *Poiēsis* not *mimesis*. Connected by the textual threads of the words the poem dances: breathes: the threads of wyrd. [*Wyrd* = Old English verbal noun formed from the verb *weorðan*, meaning 'to come to pass, to become'; cognate w/ *verse* (*n*. poetry); from the root **wer-* 'to turn, to bend'/ 'be changed'].

UTOPIAN POETICS FUNCTIONS THUS:

1. **AS POIĒSIS – PERFORMED BY THE POEM'S BECOMING**
2. **AS ANTICIPATORY ILLUMINATION OF WHAT IS NOT YET**
3. **AS EMBODIED GESTURE – SIMULTANEOUSLY PERFORMING & ANTICIPATING UTOPIA**

That is, utopian poetics simultaneously performs and anticipates the possibility of non-alienation, whilst operating within the alienation of this world. Non-alienation [communion, union, yoga] with oneself as an embodied subject and simultaneously with an/other/s is always possible to a greater extent than one can/is currently experience/ing it. Alienation [ego] persists within our experience of non-alienation [embodied intersubjectivity]. In opening up a space in which embodied and intersubjective non-alienation becomes possible between reader and writer, utopian poetics enacts the possibility of non-alienation within an alienated world. In that it is a poem/text, and not the world, it anticipates the possibility of non-alienation while recognising that non-alienation is not-yet. In short: *Utopian poetics both performs and anticipates utopia by performing the possibility of embodied intersubjectivity within the body/breath of the poem/text, the body/breath of the reader/listener and the body/breath of the writer/speaker.*

NON-ALIENATION IN UTOPIAN POETICS

Between the writer and the reader:

- *The functions of openness and multiplicity within the poem/text create a breathing space within which the writer and the reader are both active participants in the co-creation of meaning*

- *Openness and multiplicity may be generated via parataxis, juxtaposition, hesitation, use of [breathing] space within poetic form, use of [breathing] space within and between words and parts of words, a-syntactic grammar, a-teleological narrative, non-narrative, anti-narrative, the foregrounding of language's material properties/processes, the foregrounding of the material properties of the codex, or by any other generative methods*

- *The purpose of open form and multiplicity of possibility is to ensure the intersubjective agency of both writer and reader in the process of making meaning in utopian poetics*

- *It is in this co-creative process that utopian poetics performs the possibility of embodied non-alienation*

Between the writer and the source text/s

- *Additionally, the utopian poet strives to maintain a poethical, non-violent relationship with source text/s*

- *A poetics is not utopian if it employs methods or strategies of: oppression; cultural appropriation; racism; entitlement; privilege; misogyny; ableism; homophobia, transphobia or queer-phobia, in either its forms or content*

- *An ethical relationship must be maintained with one's sources as well as one's readers*

- *The utopian poet acknowledges their position within an embodied and intersubjective constellation of connections that extend horizontally, vertically and laterally through space, time and geography; this constellation includes one's sources, oneself and one's readers in a relationship performed by the writing and reading of the poem/text itself*

- *The utopian poetic is the nexus of connections performing a relationship of embodied intersubjectivity between otherwise ostensibly disparate [&/or disembodied] subjects*

- *This relationship is formed with, in, via and through the medium of language/speech and its interactions with body and breath*

- *Language, bodies & breathing, and their performance on the page or in person, are the interconnecting materials of utopian poetics*

UTOPIAN POETICS IS *NEVER* SENTIMENTAL OR NOSTALGIC

    IT DOES NOT SEEK TO CONSTRUCT FANTASY WORLDS OR

FICTIONAL BORDERS

    ALONG THE LINES OF NATIONALISM, GENDER, SEXUALITY, RACE,

OR ANY OTHER SUCH

                     EXCLUSIONARY CONSTRUCTS

UTOPIAN POETICS DOES NOT EXCLUDE

                     IT INCLUDES

          YOU ARE WELCOME

Part 2:

Asana Pranayama
Mudra Bandha

Asana

'You move. You are being moved. You are movement. Inseparably. Indefinably. Not isolatable — terms.'

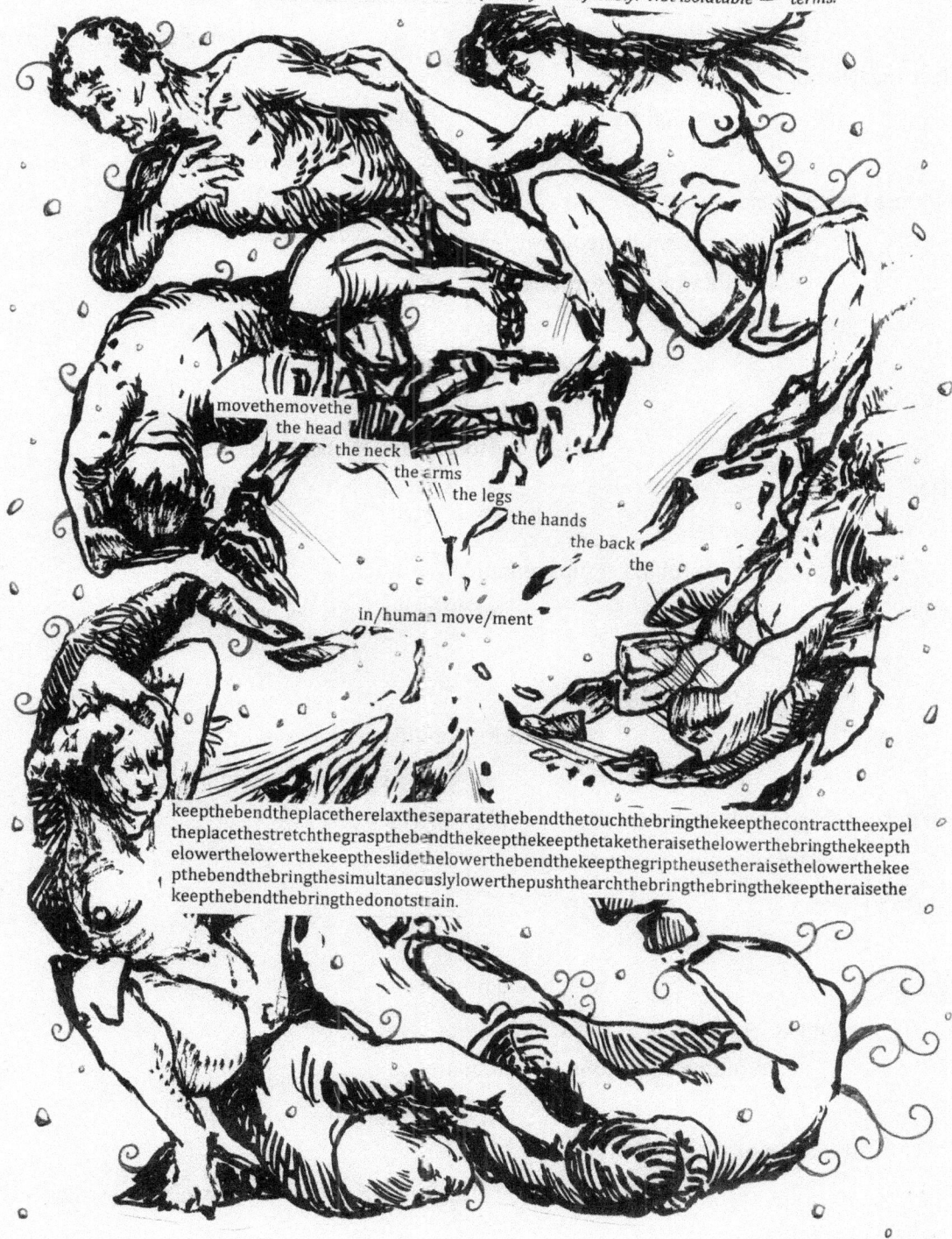

movethemovethe
the head
the neck
the arms
the legs
the hands
the back
the

in/human move/ment

keepthebendtheplacetherelaxtheseparatethebendthetouchthebringthekeepthecontracttheexpel
theplacethestretchthegraspthebendthekeepthekeepthetaketheraisethelowerthebringthekeepth
elowerthelowerthekeeptheslidethelowerthebendthekeepthegriptheusetheraisethelowerthekee
pthebendthebringthesimultaneouslylowerthepushthearchthebringthebringthekeeptheraisethe
keepthebendthebringthedonotstrain.

sthira-sukham asanam

                        breathing is movement is

                                                fundamental

                                                        of living things

st& w/ feet together or

                        slightly apart or   move   or

                                                        breathe normally

            unless the spine is

                                simultaneously the right knee

                        exhale while performing

                grip the floor

                                        bend left leg

            tilt head back

                        move   buttocks, hips & abdomen

not advised

                for people suffering

                        thighs & hips remain

inhale while   stretching the right leg back

                        bend the head

                touch the floor on either side

                                        bring forehead close as

                                                comfort.

place as if grip as if bend as if push as if stretch as if grasp as if expel as –

                back forms a ninety degree angle

            do not strain

                        do not strain

                                high blood press

            & upper trunk

                        hormone secretions   stimulate

                                                freedom of   movement

                transitional

                                                        supply chains

left door open

grace of /movement

          remove toxins

every mental knot has corresponding

          physical, muscular knot &

      vice versa

negotiate   tongue limb position

          freedom of travel

      has a corresponding

          vice versa

unrestricted

          human consciousness

               ensuring health

    kinaesthesia

cellular activity

       healthy, vigorous

    freedom of movement

            to end

                 march   2019

            block lungs

               air ways

       re/locating

     whole body

            re/move

              uncertainty

   integrating

      somato-psychically

            through the body to the mind

congestion

       the end of   free movement

     border   gridlock

            emotionally tension: block lungs

            diaphragm breathing process

     citizen of nowhere

You return & you are not   *one of*

                           them

                           they

                           treat

                           you

                           with

                           indifference.

                stiffness of

                       the body

        a subsequent accumulation

                            unresolved integration

     in the /nervous/   system

                   registration   migrants

       work & live in

                    temporary suspension

    emotional muscles

                 control all the joints

                       strengthen the

      narrative of imperial white supremacy

                supply chains

    block lungs

               stiffness &   kinamnesia

                    increase friction

              imprisonment in nation

       states   inconsistent

   divorce

      arrest

hammer out

       breathing is

          movement is

              fundamental

                life process

take back control

        negotiate

          extending

              rights to people

freedom to travel

          versatility

     transforming   force

                 oxygenate blood

                    to the brain

                          as if

individuals could

    align their own

        internal structures

           to resonate

               w/ cosmic light   or

embodied into cellular memory

       increasing mental clarity

          reproductive, circulatory, respiratory

              & digestive systems

            release

dormant energy

     become light

           creative

  biorhythms of body

       in positions that

                   cultivate

Pranayama
'the HEART, by way of the BREATH, to the LINE'

percussions   repercussions
              breathing /forcing
                  breathing /forcing
                        breathing /for
                forced exhalation
                          hex
                hexhalation
   hexhexhalation
              forced exhalation
       excess   excess   excess
                              mucous
percussions   repercussions
                  perception   pain   reverses normal
              contraction forceful
                        lungs
                          both nostrils
                      hexhale   hexhale
percussions   re/percussions
                  vulnerable
                    suffered
                \\despite repeated
hexhalation
              hexhalation
                      judicial instruction\\
             morbidity mortality "publichealthemergency"
percussions   repercussions
             hyoid   thyroid nitrogen   dioxide
                larynx   pharynx   excess
                      exhalation

limits

phonation

worst affected

Birmingham   Brixton

inhalation

friction

mucous

mortality

percussion   repercussion

hexhale hexhale hexhale hexhale

hex   hex   hex

Mudra

'I suddenly see that the gesture of a hand could be a poem –
like the mark it might leave impressed in a surface.'

– Scott Thurston, *Reverses Heart's Reassembly*

the Sanskrit word *mudra* is translated as 'gesture' or 'attitude'

a mudra may involve the whole body

or it may be a simple   hand position

fingerstouching

inside   thumb

I offer flowers.

touch the root   of each

mudra: = *mud* (delight, pleasure) + *dravay*, *dru* (to draw forth)

chin mudra is consciousness

when the palms face upward in *chin mudra*, the chest area is opened: up.

relaxed   hand

index   finger and thumb

the practitioner may experience this as a sensation of lightness and receptivity

hasta (hand) mudras

which join the thumb & index finger

psycho-neural finger locks

loop of energy

emitted by hands

back into body

mudras manipulate prana in much the same way that energy in the form of light or   sound
waves is diverted by a mirror or a cliff face. cliff edge.

                        while

                              naked power   grab   by ministers
to   straighten   index fingers
                              and

                                    take back

                                                control

                                                      so that

            slightly apart.the unity

                              two   fold

                                    will of the british people

gives

                  the ultimate   finger

                                    and

                                    rapidly leads to internalization.

thumb and index finger tend   to separate more easily

                                    when body awareness

                                                is lost

B&ha

theSanskritwordb&hameansholdtightenlock

extremerestraintmechanistackleillegalim
migrantlockthemfirmintopositiondetentin
tensthepressureappliedtightagainstchestin
creasedheartrate&tenseheavybreathemp
tylungs&beingabusedwhatevdurationhu
mancostlongretentstrainsheartincreased
paintensioninspineremovefrombritainin
tensifpressureappliedtoneckcarotidarter
iessurvivalinstinctrustytoiletnobed&urge
toprocreategranthispreventtheflowofpra
nadonotinhaledeliberatecreate'hostileen
vironment'governdigestion&metabolise
foodbeneficialincorporateanxiet&tension
strainheartifsuffocatetargethomelesseun
ationalstodeportapplypressuretoperineal/
vaginallockmasterdugintomyskinpulled
backdownkneesinfirmcontactw/floor
lockpranasinpartic&redirectforpurpo
seoftensifypressureincreasedetentionof
humanexistentinhumantreatmentfalsein
tenteunationalsinbritainlockthemintoposi
textremetraumanotcompliantbacklock
otherestraintpsychicknotspreventthusim
pedeinyarlswoodimmigrateremovecen
trebedfordshiredetentions&enforcedexpo
feucitizensfromukrisesharpsincestressanx
ietangerhardentonetowardnationalitmen
talhealth&gendlockthemfirmlyinanxiet
depresspstdprimalnrgretainifdurabeincrea
sethenwherethefearofdeath&homeofficeim
migratcompliant&enforcement(ICE)team

Part 3:
Three Rituals for
Theresa Hak Kyung Cha

ghostword sembles itself

        antiphony then past

                the synonym each satisfactory

            word approaching

                  still unarticulated   unresolved

                                                nomenclature

            resembles utopian tension

                in other words

time release much

        with ritual

            byword notation absence

whether occurred

            begins more rehearsals   more

        charting All map One

                least that no documenting keep

                    appease. follow

. equivalence

        would byname

                unconcluded exile

the ghostword dissembles

            itself unhoused

        cemetery   tomb

            death would /never

                could /continue to /live

            without /ceasing

                    .search the words

events that have occurred or are to come

                    display before

                voyeur.voyeur.

        antiphony to follow

                begins more rehearsals

pain/less translating provisionally

        metaphor

          absence ending

                the ghostword sembles

equivalence   would appease

          satisfactory byword

            translating memory

                  antiphony release with

              sooth

whether translating more rehearsals more absence synonym

       feeling equivalence charting All notation

               keep documenting

               originary point/ here

       ritual weather begins metaphor

    equivalence would byname

       the ghostword sembles itself

                     merely

            intimate

           a kind of

               remembering

             equivalence

        in other words

             reverberations of

               ourselves

         misrecognized

             nearing hearing

           evocable

             blueness at the heart

               still unarticulated

        music it is literature is book

            yielding

             yielding

        quiet phantoms for the root

   search. the words

            i wonder /who

has brought /the

flowers

re/as/sembled paris

22 june 1976

rain by the tomb

/ tristan tzara

sitting in

montparnasse i wonder

word approaching intimate

goes towar

the unsayable

of becoming

another

incompletion

re/vocable

in other words

Not Yet

urge to correspond

what has just been

said in other words

creaking ice

must be crossed

in intelligible worlds

human voice hearing /nearing

itself

merely intimate

being-missing

in other words semblance this moonlit landscape more

or less lived

incognito

misrecognized

equivalence

fluidity, darkness

                              so that nothing
                    shone enough for
                              absolute crisis
              ir/revocable
                    citizenship in intelligible worlds
                              exile
                    at least despair
                                   remains
                located
                         in other words
                                        as this moment
                              the possibility
                              hears itself
              revolutionary /serpent
                         constantly undermining
                              translation
        reassembled in other words
                                   still /unarticulated
                    death would never
                              not yet vocable
              concurrent with the
                         strangely weary and obscure
                              originary point here
                                        the unavoidable end
                              whispered every possibility
                              of evocation
              blackout
                    what has just been said
                                   presently wavering
                         homesickness
                              want to vomit
        absolute crisis hears itself unsayableresemblance
                              verbal/reassemblage

apocalyptic kernel

          reclaiming

           itself as answer

            antiphony to follow

     weather simile metaphor ghostword

search the words

   for the root

          the words or vocables

   reciting-to-oneself

     paris 1976

        death would never

   silence the stars   by.name

  in other words shudder   disassembled

     at the heart

       a brief notation

      abolish real time write

       without ceasing

invocable   a word   is

       approaching

       approximating

       intimat/ing

      semblance

       resemblance

  synonym ghostword

    displace/ment

      exiled

    nomenclature

   entire silence reclaiming

      the inconstruable

purely/   as question

   unknowing

     what has just

      been said

                                        so that
                                                    nothing
                                        located
            so far away so   near
                            more or
                                    less in other
                        human voice at least despair
                beyond the lettering
                                incompletion
                                            re-vocable
                    unavoidable end of
        kernel reverberating
                                    in other   words
                yielding. yielding
                                provisionally intimate
                    more or less located
                            urge to correspond

Cha's Hands, 1979

quiver
quaver
quick
sense
hands
aware
SING
fingers long and
slender
elliptical
lunula
[no] scars,[no] marks
dimples
the knuckle
middle finger,
both hands
reaching across
the typewriter
keys
curled right fingers
rest;
left fingers
oblique
straddle
right
thumb on
space
left thumb in space
raise sinew from
left ring finger
wrist
light lifting ridge
left
index
knuckle
no keys
have been pressed
you are
relaxed
choosing
to identify
your
self as
two hands
typing is
who you are
typing
a type of
who you will be
who you have been
who you were
who you are here
marks you
make

on life
you
type
the words forming
       in space
you type
the words
She says to herself
if she were
able to write
she could
continue
to
live
your hands
the keys
writing
writing
inscribing
on air
inscribing
on your
muscles
tendons
joints
memory
the keys
that form
the words
impossible
to write
and writing
in
words
innovative or
resistant
you
participant
in the writing
experiment
modification
corporeal
performance
implicated
involvement
the act of
writing
signifying
parsing
altering
sculpting
your moving body
in the act
of writing

measuring
       st/utter
iterating &
reiterating
kinaesthetic
experience
falter
decisions
innovative or
resistant
trace
your gestures
type
inscription
embodied gesturing
individual
implicated
, yes, resistance
rejection of the
routine and
ambiguous
yielding
sensory experience
simultaneously
written upon
and
writing
if she would
write
without
ceasing
your fingers
motion
through
all you have
known and
have
forgotten
to inscribe
your words
yourself
fleeting
and
always
the difference
resisting
gesturing
indicating
your hands
your words
inscribed in space
written in air
inscribing &
incorporate

infinite imperative

to

turn the directions
learn the directions
burn the directions

you

turn the seasons
start facing south
window to valley
curtain to   colden to
calder
colden to window to
curtain to calder
colden to calder
to curtain
to valley
to colden to face to window to calder
to season to start to turn the

ly breathe: silence

you

turn facing north
to slack to hebden   water
colden to hebd
to slacken to
north
to valley to window to water
slacken face to
season turn to
curtain out   the colder

breathe: silence
fire
log to burn to
turn to learn to
smithy the seasons   faster
to face to burn to log to turn to
smithereen
to falter
to valley to vale to
window to wail to slacken fire to

breathe: silence

you

west to face

you

east to easter
book to quester
wall to turn to fog to winder
rise to cold to hept on stall to veil to
face to future
to gift to wing to blister linger
seas on turn to duster

breathe: silence

synovial
fluid

breathe: silence

distil   extend   breath

distillation extending breath to its utmost pure to purer

you

stand a column
of ~~white~~ lustre
atoned with tears
restored in breath

stand a river
breathing
silence
breathing
rhythm
deeper

turn

cerebrospinal
fluid (C.S.F.)

arterial blood

cellular fluid

interstitial fluid

venous blood

FIGURE 29

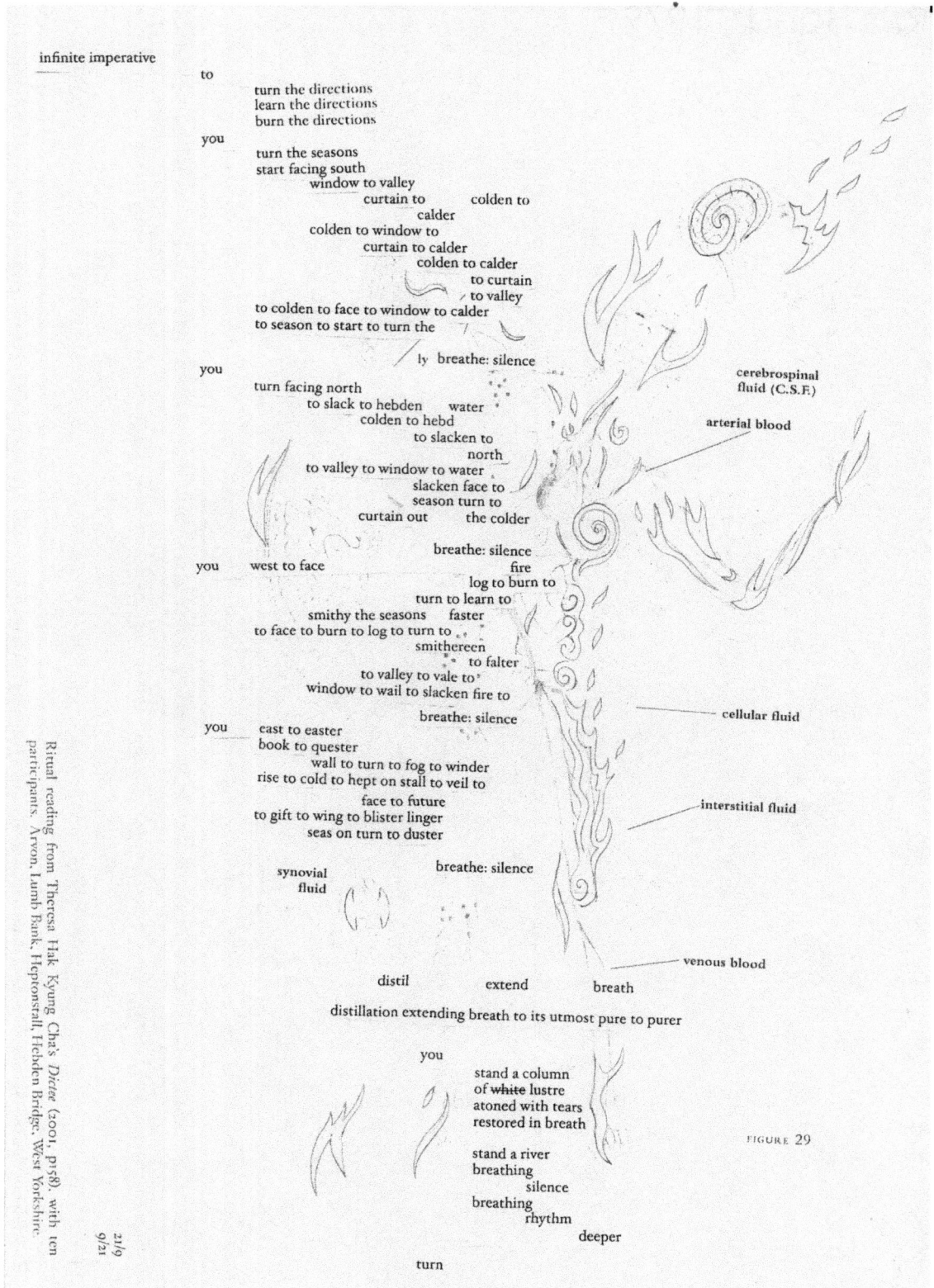

Ritual reading from Theresa Hak Kyung Cha's *Dictee* (2001, p158), with ten participants, Arvon, Lumb Bank, Heptonstall, Hebden Bridge, West Yorkshire.

21/9
9/21

Part 4:
Movement &
Meditation

& how to metabolise this
        & how to & how to
            & how to
metabolise this
            & how to
            & how //
                & how to
                    metabolise this
                    & how to & how to
            & how to   metabolisethis
                    &howto
                    &howto
                    &howto
                        meta b lie/s this
                            &howto
                                &howt]

        //this >>   chlorine washed >>//con
    stant era/sure / re/place/ment
                        do[u]sed w/
                        hormones
                all /or/ nothing /in/digestible
                        /phr/
                riddle w/ toxins
                you say you
                        \
                lentilsasparagus
                ex/treme fat/igue &
                eco/nom/ic ex/clusion
                    so poor as
                    to be unl/awful

>>global/

body/fascism/

de/crease /di/versity

in/crease /ris/k

residues of steroids

brexfist

&howto   &howto   &howto   &howto

&howto   [meta]b/lies this   &howto

&howto

&howto metabolisethis

antibiotics as routine/ feed

irritable/bowel

globalised/growth

chlorine immersion >>>all \or\ nothing\\\\

palm oil plantations

break\fast

processed

&howtoo&

&howtoo&

&howtoo&

endless escalation

self-possession

ext\\in\guished

pre\biotic quick \fix

compared w/ placebo

no point \arrival

: transit

bit /like >>The Lost Boys

chemical-treat/d/GMO/d/chlorine-wash/d/

&howto metabolise this

America\n\Dream\Die\t

race to >>th/ bottom]

dehydrated&contracted

cntrctd&dhdrtd

cntrctd

cntrct/d

cntrct

&howto metabolise this

poison/in/ yr body   poison/in/ yr plant/s

enhanc/d global trade

binge-eat-hormone-inject/d-car/s

break\\ down

running \slow\

living \in\ dark \

climate

&howto&howto

my voice

is /my

password

my /voice

ismy

passwrd

=== myvoice

is

&howto

&how/to

&how\too

myvoice

&howto

&howto

&hwto

myvoice

&howto

ins/ex/subs/res/ist /on //facts

read you /think you/

say you\ become

indi/gest\ible/phr\

&howto

&howto

&howto

&howtometabolise

&howtometabolise

&speak\same

&speaksame

&speak/same

=========la<<<

&probioticking is a verb&

flow-staccato-chaos-lyrical-stillness

Deeper breathing
through arm-movement.

flow of breath

through body

exhaled as

beingness

sweat-scented

must

arcs

hips

feet

arms up,
Stronger
Grounding

feet

flow

breath

singing

ecstatic
YELL
of presence

hereness

is

us

in room

from insides

depth
of presence

beneath
surface

describing

V

describing

in communion

with smooth

oak

floor

describing

describing

canto

bodies

arrives

announcing

arms down,
lighter
upwards
experience

in communion w/

in rhythm

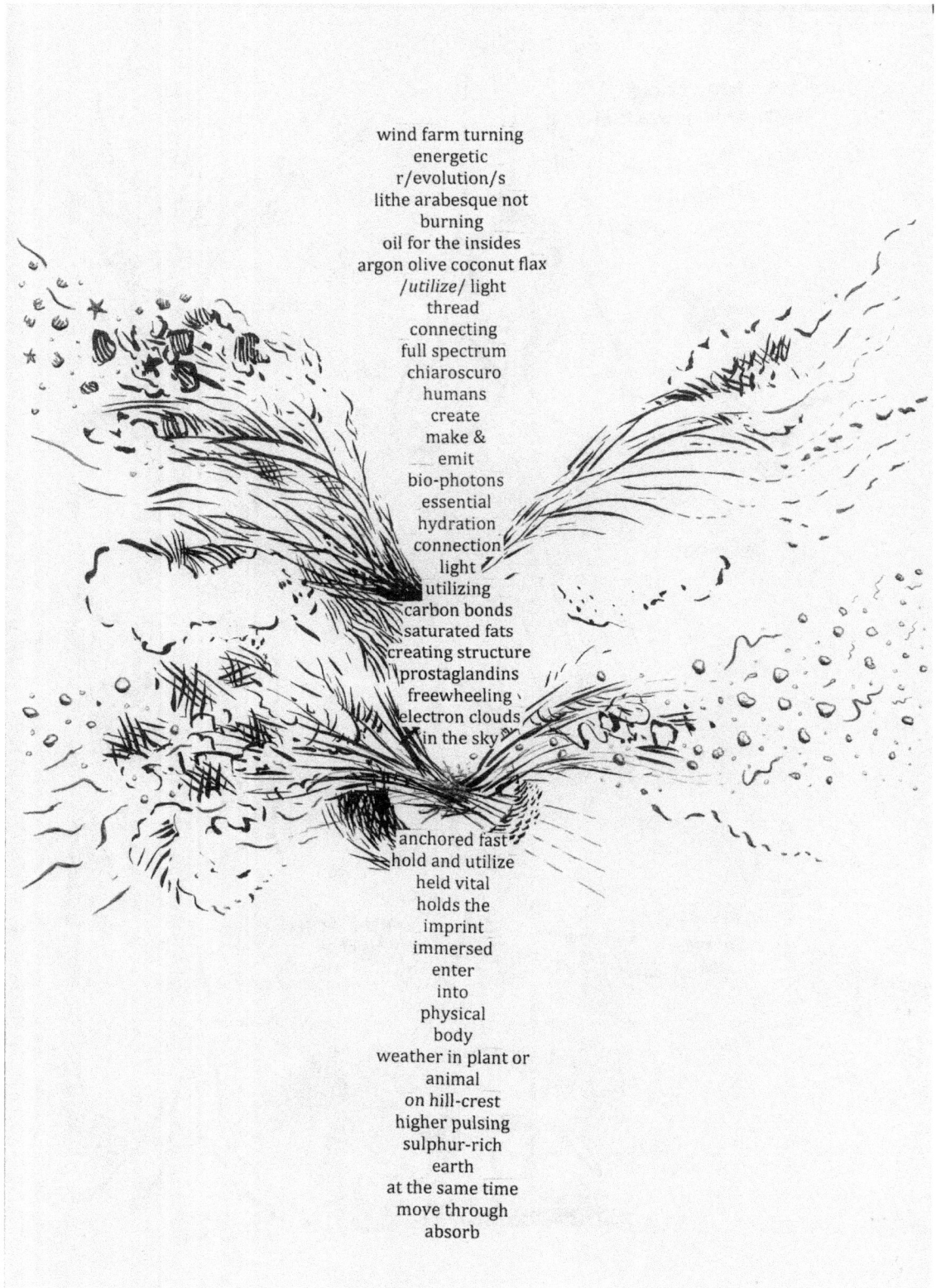

wind farm turning
energetic
r/evolution/s
lithe arabesque not
burning
oil for the insides
argon olive coconut flax
/utilize/ light
thread
connecting
full spectrum
chiaroscuro
humans
create
make &
emit
bio-photons
essential
hydration
connection
light
utilizing
carbon bonds
saturated fats
creating structure
prostaglandins
freewheeling
electron clouds
in the sky

anchored fast
hold and utilize
held vital
holds the
imprint
immersed
enter
into
physical
body
weather in plant or
animal
on hill-crest
higher pulsing
sulphur-rich
earth
at the same time
move through
absorb

rhythm of a living

Western society is
>>> chron/ic/ally
>>>> sleep
> deprived

'being potentially
>> present'
lose >>> ability
>> to hold
> elect/(r)on ///
>> clouds

- what is physical
>> *light*
inside
> *yr body?*

the way that
> DNA
> is read
>> or
'transcribed'

> yr body's language
dimly lit
>> within the cell
age old age old age
> & in(es)capable

endless

    feedback

        looping

undulating

    on-off-on-off-on-off-off-off-off-on-on-on-on-on-on-on-on

           cycles

    linked to

        retina

secret/e

    hormones

        activity

           of blood

all rise & fall

    all rise

        & fall

        all

        rise

           &

        fall

           all

               rise

                    &

                        f/all

bright lights

    before

bedtime

    [rhythm of   a living]

move back

    into the cell

at night

        continual / mental

        twilight

        not

        in tune

        melatonin tone in tone intone

        yr body language

        serotonin toning toning toning toning

        yr body language

        dopamine

        yr body language

        norepinephrine

        yr body language

        pinoline

        yr body language

        DNA yr body language

        DMT yr body language

        [yr body's language]

dancing

    to the rhythm

        (of the day/night /cycle)

        sense the sun

        on back

           of new

        anxiety

stress manifests

    inside our cell[v]s

        potassium magnesium

        sodium & calcium

                endless undulation

feeding back

    cycles

          suprachiasmatic

    cycles

      night

        & day

          cycles

            connect

              pineal

[rhythm of a   living]

    high levels of

      (the) blue(/s)

        light(s)

          diminish

            [//?~~natural~~?//]

v /in a

    dimly /lit

      office

      ng [it]"

network of clocks

in cells

controlling   bodies

in dark

unexpected

dis-ease

spreading

powerful

influen/zes

long term health

consequences

toxicity

re/membered

over-ride

over ride

override

overwrite

companies// launching

increasing ra[n]ge >>

[of products]

active in almost every

time-keeping-keeping-time-keeping

machinery

jet lag >feels

all rise

    & falls

        light re/vision

          & sound

            that radical

              slowly trickles

RHYTHM FOR A LIVING

    encodes a protein

        rhythm for a living

          respect the outsideinsideoutsidein

        rhythm for a living

                            begin

                             with/in

rhythm of (a) living

    syn/chron/us

      w/

    earth's

      re/sound/ing

        r/e/volution/s/

Guided Meditation
for Maggie O'Sullivan

imagine you're singing

several north seasing

light up / your spine

>> ulular >>   voicing >>

(schumannly resonance

accessible only

/ by /

frac/tu/ring /

through feet

standing on shoulders

of frackfielding workers

lungs / go down /

// centring //

earth's Many Root-

Song

you

balance

on /your

quietly breather

inviting

these asthmas,

silicosis / notice

your chest /

(full congester

retch/ed/ly

gas/per

exhale

      inhaler

are you lying [or]

  standing

//on the shoulders//

strong root connecter /ing

    un/hunger

        all part

            blink eyes as water

    , between,

quieten breath/er/ing >> >>

            inshale [&] exshaling

    several north seas/on

               voice //

        debatering

              roots

    >voice rootles>>

frack/field   worker   slung

    \only hope

      this democracy

   only hope

     shale gas\

   imagine:

oil well in Balcombe

        light up your spine

shale gas / in Lancashire//

        human re/semblance

//accessible only / by /

      frac/king/cyng/sing/

its root / is /

/ &also& / at the same time

a prophesy >

notice your chest

/ voice congester /

: standing on shoulders

of [Liverpool] future

roots begin sprouter

/same nonsense/

you balance /on

notice /

you're chesting

touch earth

deeper rooting

- and soon -

these asthmas / silicosis

not sure

/ notice /

only hope

shale gas

[singing]

voice roots beginning :

edgewordering

quiet breath in/viting

dis / re / sembl / ance / ing

voice roots: beginning–

blinker / your eyes stay
underground /
clinched in deep soil i'm
not sure
what democracy
this country
we paying

blink /your eyes open
blink –
you're singing
ulular / ululing
music of presence /of/
death in the voicing
unspeakably / emptying
silence of /
prophecy

imaginely
dancering
rootering
seasinging
shale gas
sprout
in you chestering
lung
in you voicering
speak
nonsensing
sap
are you
nothing
less
: : rise again
standing

= blink your eyes opening:

blink

//splitly voicing//

ulular ululing

rise again

unduling

schumannly resoning

rise again

prophesing

Notes:

Part 1: Writing Utopia Now

1. *Atha yogānuśāsanam (Patanjali's Yoga Sutras*, 1:1)

2. *Tat twam asi (Chandogya Upanishad* 6:12-14)

3. *Wyrd, weorðan, verse, *wer- (The Oxford Dictionary of English Etymology*: Oxford, 1966)

4. 'Anticipatory illumination' and 'not yet' (Bloch, Ernst [1988] *The Utopian Function of Art and Literature*, trans. Jack Zipes (ed.) and Frank Mecklenberg. Cambridge, MA: MIT Press)

5. 'Poethical' (Retallack, Joan [2003] *The Poethical Wager*. Berkeley, CA: University of California Press)

6. A version of 'Writing Utopia Now' was published in the 'Utopian Acts' Special Issue of *Studies in Arts and Humanities Journal*, May 2019. My thanks to the editors, Katie Stone and Raphael Kabo.

Part 2: Asana Pranayama Mudra Bandha

Part 2, '*Asana Pranayama Mudra Bandha*' writes through the yoga manual *Asana Pranayama Mudra Bandha* by Swami Satyananda Saraswati (Yoga Publications Trust, Munger, Bihar, India. Fourth edition [2008]) and various contemporary news articles published in *The Guardian* in 2017.

The poems '*Pranayama*', '*Mudra*' and '*B&ha*' were first published as 'Three Yoga Poems' in Burning House Press, November 2018. My thanks to guest editor, paul hawkins.

Asana

1. Collage includes an image from *Living Breath: From Inside Out* (2006) by Angela Farmer and Victor van Kooten, Berkeley, CA: Ganesha Press, plus doodles by Joe Evans.

2. Italicised quotations (with the exception of italicised Sanskrit) are from Theresa Hak Kyung Cha's *DICTEE* (2001 [1982]), Berkeley, CA: University of California Press.

Pranayama

'the HEART, by way of the BREATH, to the LINE': Charles Olson, Projective Verse (1950).

Mudra

1. 'I suddenly see that the gesture of a hand could be a poem –
    like the mark it might leave impressed in a surface.'
    Scott Thurston, *Reverses Heart's Reassembly* (2011), London: Veer

2. 'I offer flowers' from 'Offering Flowers' in *Technicians of the Sacred* (2017) ed. Jerome Rothenberg,
    Oakland, CA: University of California Press, p71.

Part 3: Three Rituals for Theresa Hak Kyung Cha

ghostword sembling

1. Reconstructed reading: Theresa Hak Kyung Cha, *Dictee* p140 & 'the sound is a dripping faucet'
    from *Exilée and Temps Morts* ([2009], ed. Constance M. Lewallen, Berkeley, CA: University of California
    Press) p134; Ernst Bloch 'The shape of the Inconstruable Question' from *Spirit of Utopia* ([2000], trans.
    Anthony A. Nassar, Stanford, CA: Stanford University Press).

    On 22nd June 1976, Theresa Hak Kyung Cha sat by the tomb of Tristan Tzara in Montparnasse
    Cemetery, Paris, listening to the rain. She wrote about this experience in a journal entry
    beginning with the words 'the sound is a dripping faucet'. This gesture instigates a cut-up
    practice to disassemble and reassemble some of Cha's words, creating the opportunity to
    liberate some of her vocabulary from the poetic structures she creates in her writing and hear
    her words with fresh resonance. Reading and collaging these words with found vocabulary
    from Bloch's *Spirit of Utopia* gestures towards the (in)articulation of the unsayable, or the
    utopian, which I identify as an element of the utopian poetics that drives Cha's text works.

2. 'nomenclature' from *Restless Continent* by Aja Couchois Duncan (2016), Brooklyn, NY: Litmus Press.

3. Variations on the word 'vocable' have at least one tendril of their root in Jerome Rothenberg's
    original (1967) preface to *Technicians of the Sacred*. Rothenberg, J. (2017). *Technicians of the
    Sacred*. Oakland, CA: University of California Press, pp. xxx – xxxix.

Cha's Hands, 1979

Ekphrastic response to the photograph by James Cha printed in *The Dream of the Audience: Theresa Hak
Kyung Cha (1951-1982)* (2001), ed. Constance M. Lewallen, Berkeley, CA: University of California Press,
(n.p.). Includes quotations from *Dictee*, p141 + writes through some of the vocabulary and ideas from
Agency and Embodiment: Performing Gestures/Producing Culture (2009), Carrie Noland, Harvard University
Press.

infinite imperative

21/9
9/21
Ritual reading from Theresa Hak Kyung Cha's *Dictee*, p158, with ten participants. Arvon, Lumb Bank, Heptonstall, Hebden Bridge, West Yorkshire.

A version of this poem was originally published in *Zarf*, Issue 10, December 2017. My thanks to callie gardner.

Collage includes an image from *Yoga Mind, Body & Spirit: a Return to Wholeness* (2000), Donna Farhi, New York, NY: Holt Paperbacks; plus hand-drawn illustrations by Joe Evans.

Part 4: Movement & Meditation

Poems in this section write through Barbara Wren's *Cellular Awakening: How Your Body Holds and Creates Light* ([2009], London: Hay House) and various contemporary news articles published in *The Guardian* in 2017.

& how to

1. This poem is developed from an originally improvised sound poem performed at *Hákarl 24* in Brighton, a 24-hour continuous improvisation with 12 participants in July 2017. Sources for this poem include various news articles, notes from a conversation with a friend about her experience of living on a fruit farm in Ecuador, overheard snippets from a telephone call, Barbara Wren's *Cellular Awakening*.

2. This poem borrows and adapts the line 'the undigestible phrase' from Lorine Niedecker's 'a country's economics sick' (Lorine Niedecker: Collected Works [2002], Berkeley, CA: University of California Press, p86).

flow – staccato – chaos – lyrical – stillness

Collage includes an image from *Living Breath: From Inside Out* (2006) by Angela Farmer and Victor van Kooten, Berkeley, CA: Ganesha Press.

wind farm turning

1. Collage includes an image from *Living Breath: From Inside Out* (2006) by Angela Farmer and Victor van Kooten, Berkeley, CA: Ganesha Press, plus doodles by Joe Evans.

2. A version of this poem was first published in *The Projectionist's Playground*, Issue 4, December 2017. My thanks to Julius Smit.

rhythm of a living

1. This poem writes through found text from *Yoga Anatomy* by Leslie Kaminoff (2007, Human Kinetics), *Recreating the Psychoactive Forest: Nutrition for Natural Consciousness* by Holly Paige (2010), *Cellular Awakening* by Barbara Wren (2009) and 'Western Society is Chronically Sleep Deprived' by Hannah Devlin in *The Guardian* 6 October 2017.

2. 'being potentially present' is from Richard Foreman 'Trying to be Centered … On the Circumference' in *The L=A=N=G=U=A=G=E Book* (1984), ed. Bruce Andrews and Charles Bernstein, Carbondale and Edwardsville: Southern Illinois University Press, p50.

3. *'what is physical light inside yr body?'* is borrowed and adapted from Mei-mei Berssenbrugge's 'Endocrinology' in *Out of Everywhere 2: Linguistically Innovative Poetry by Women in North America & the UK* (2015) ed. Emily Critchley, Hastings: Reality Street, p26.

Guided Meditation: for Maggie O'Sullivan

1. This poem was workshopped and developed with the guidance of Harriet Tarlo and Scott Thurston at Arvon Lumb Bank in September 2017. I am grateful for their guidance and the friendship and support of everyone on the 'Experimental Poetry: Playing with Form and Language' course. The poem was completed in *Our Humblest of Pleasures*, vegan café, Hebden Bridge, which was joyfully recommended to me by Maggie O'Sullivan when she came to read her poetry at Lumb Bank. I am humbly thankful for making this connection and I am grateful to Maggie for her subsequent kindnesses to me.

2. This poem is developed from a sound collage including clips from the following sources:

    Caroline Lucas at Fracking Protest Balcombe:
    www.youtube.com/watch?v=5ZrINcEnNZE

    Fracking Debate 'How dare you lie on national tv?':
    www.youtube.com/watch?v=v9w3RBLf7D4

    Fracking Debate on Newsnight:
    www.youtube.com/watch?v=v9w3RBLf7D4

    Rooting & Grounding Guided Meditation - Suzanne Wright Yoga:
    www.youtube.com/watch?v=tx5ZhNYK1Dw

    Gaia Healing Earth's Frequency 7.8hz Music (Schumann Resonance):
    www.youtube.com/watch?v=k1GUN0k7Y9I

3. This poem was first published online in *Adjacent Pineapple*, Issue 2, 2017. My thanks to Colin J. Herd.

4. 'earth's Many Root- /Song 'quoted from OF MUTABILITY

5. 'its root is also at the same time a prophesy' is borrowed and adapted from BOG ASPHODEL SONG Both from *In the House of the Shaman* (1993), Maggie O'Sullivan, Hastings: Reality Street.

9 781912 211432